Copyright © 2o20 by Katrina W. Paul -All rights reserved.

No part of this book may be reproduced or transmitted in any form or by any means, electronic or mechanical, including photocopying and recording, or by any information storage and retrieval system, without permission in writing from the publisher. This is a work of fiction. Names, places, characters and incidents are either the product of the author's imagination or are used fictitiously, and any resemblance to any actual persons, living or dead, organizations, events or locales is entirely coincidental. The unauthorized reproduction or distribution of this copyrighted work is ilegal.

Please note the information contained within this document is for educational and entertainment purposes only. All effort has been executed to present accurate, up to date, reliable, complete information. No warranties of any kind are declared or implied. Readers acknowledge that the author is not engaged in the rendering of legal, financial, medical, or professional advice. The content within this book has been derived from various sources. Please consult a licensed professional before attempting any techniques outlined in this book. By reading this document, the reader agrees that under no circumstances is the author responsible for any losses, direct or indirect, that are incurred as a result of the use of the information contained within this document, including, but not limited to, errors, omissions, or inaccuracies.

CONTENTS

INTRODUCTION 4
ASIAN COUNTRIES AND THEIR CUISINE 5
ADVANTAGES OF ASIAN MEALS AND CUISINE 6
CHICKEN RECIPES 7
    1-Flavorful Tandoori Chicken 7
    2-Stir Fry Chicken 8
    3-Spicy Chicken Wings 9
    4-Delicious Chicken Thighs 10
    5-Crispy Chicken Wings 11
    6-BBQ Chicken Wings 12
    7-Lemon Honey Chicken 13
    8-Korean Chicken Wings 14
    9-Tangy Chicken 15
    10-Sriracha Chicken Wings 16
MEAT RECIPES 17
    11-Simple Air Fried Pork Chunks 17
    12-Chinese Pork Roast 18
    13-Spicy Korean Pork 19
    14-Tasty BBQ Beef 20
    15-Crispy Pork Chops 21
    16-Ginger Garlic Beef 22
    17-Spicy Lamb 23
    18-Beef Kabab 24
    19-Crispy Grilled Pork 25
    20-Flavorful Lamb Steak 26
FISH & SEAFOOD RECIPES 27
    21-Garlic Lemon Shrimp 27
    22-Salmon Patties 28
    23-Shrimp with Sauce 29
    24-Honey Soy Salmon 30
    25-Tasty Asian Shrimp 31
    26-Healthy Salmon Patties 32
    27-Sriracha Salmon 33
    28-Ginger Garlic Shrimp 34
    29-Lemon Chili Shrimp 35
    30-Crispy Coconut Shrimp 36
SIDE DISHES 37
    31-Sweet Potato Bites 37
    32-Crispy Cauliflower Florets 38
    33-Banana Chips 39
    34-Broccoli with Pine Nuts 40
    35-Garlic Cauliflower Florets 41
VEGETARIAN & TOFU RECIPES 42
    36-Roasted Broccoli with Peanuts 42
    37-Garlic Brussels sprouts 43

- 38-Delicious Air Fried Tofu...44
- 39-Lemon Garlic Broccoli Florets...45
- 40-Crispy Tofu..46

DESSERTS & SNACKS...47
- 41-Delicious Chinese Doughnuts..47
- 42-Sweet & Crisp Bananas..48
- 43-Banana Muffins...49
- 44-Easy Blueberry Muffins...50
- 45- Spicy Mix Nuts...51

KETO ASIAN RECIPES..52
- 46-Healthy Air Fried Okra..52
- 47-Sausage Meatballs...53
- 48-Chicken Meatballs..54
- 49-Delicious Chicken Kebabs..55
- 50-Easy Chinese Chicken Wings...56

INTRODUCTION

An air fryer is one of the healthiest ways of cooking, without using too much fat for cooking. Compared to deep frying, an air fryer needs a lesser amount of fat. It also helps to reduce calories and minimize potentially harmful compounds from your food. An air fryer cooks food by circulating hot air around the food like a convection mechanism.

Air fryers are now very popular in many Asian countries. There are various different types of Air fryer available on the market. The most popular is a basket type air fryer, it requires less oil compared to other air fryers. You can bake cakes using baking pan accessories and also cook curries in it.

In this book, you will learn various types of Asian meals and their cuisine. It includes 50 different recipes for Air Fryers in different cooking styles like Chinese style, Korean style, Indian style, Japanese style and so on.

ASIAN COUNTRIES AND THEIR CUISINE

Indian cuisine:
Most of the diverse cuisines found in India are due to their different religions, culture, soil, and climate etc. The traditional food of India is famous worldwide due to its ingredients, herbs, spices and different cooking styles. In India, there are mainly two cooking styles divided by their regions one is south Indian and another is north Indian cuisine.

Indian cuisines have their unique and strong flavor come from spices, herbs and nutritious ingredients like leafy vegetables, legume, grains, and fruits. Many of the ingredients have medicinal properties like cloves, turmeric is antiseptic, and ginger is good for digestion. A well balanced Indian food is categorized into six tastes such as spicy, sweet, sour, bitter, astringent and salty. The use of numerous combined spices is the secret of Indian recipes.

Japanese cuisine:
Japanese cuisine offers a variety of regional and seasonal dishes. Many of the Japanese restaurants are specialized in single types of dishes and some offer a variety of dishes. Traditional Japanese dishes are basically based on rice with miso soup and other dishes consist of cooked vegetables in broth, pickled vegetables, and fish. Seafood is common in Japanese cuisine, often grilled but also serve raw in sushi. Sushi is one of the popular Japanese dishes, basically raw fish with rice. Some other popular Japanese dishes are rice dishes, noodle dishes, meat dishes, seafood dishes, soybean dishes, nabe dishes, yoshoku dishes etc.

Korean cuisine:
Korean foods are based on rice, meat, vegetables, noodles, and tofu. Korean cuisine offers various types of side dishes like broiled beef, bean paste soup, cabbage (kimchi), fish and steamed vegetables. Kimchi is basically a fermented vegetable dish made up of Korean radish, napa cabbage which is highly seasoned with garlic, pepper etc. Most of the Korean dishes are simple especially known for their odors and pungent flavors.

Chinese Cuisine:
Chinese cuisine is one of the most popular cuisines in the world. Chinese cuisines are famous for its aroma, taste, color, and appearance. Chinese cooking doesn't use too much oil for frying purpose; they use healthy substance in large quantities. Chinese foods are very unique and traditional; rice is the favorite grain in south China. Bread, noodles, sorghum, corn millet, vegetables, cabbage, and tofu are used in the Chinese diet. A typical Chinese home meal contains boiled rice, steamed fish, stir-fried pork with vegetables and soup.

Vietnamese cuisine:
Vietnamese dishes are popular for their distinctive flavor. It includes most common ingredients like soy sauce, fish sauce, rice, fresh herbs, shrimp paste, bean sauce, fruits vegetables and fresh herbs like lemongrass, lime, and kaffir lime leaves. Vietnamese foods are considered as the healthiest cuisine worldwide. Herbs and fresh vegetables are essential in many Vietnamese dishes, broth, and soup-based dishes are very common in Vietnamese cuisine. Vietnamese cuisines are usually colorful and arranged in eye-pleasing manners in serving dishes.

Pilipino cuisine:
Most of the countries have a culture to eat food three times a day but in the Philippines, the rules are different they eat food six times a day. Lechon is a popular festive dish, lechon is suckling pig in Spanish. It is a whole pig roasted over charcoal for many hours. Lechon is considering as a national dish of the Philippines. The city of Cebu is one of the most famous places to eat famous dish lechon.

Burmese cuisine:
Burmese cuisines are inspired by Chinese, Thai and Indian cuisine. Mohinga is a traditional dish in Burmese cuisine and it is also a national dish of Burma. Seafood is used as a common ingredient in Burma cities. Burmese cuisine also includes verities of salads like rice noodles, rice, vermicelli, glass noodles, ginger, potato, kaffir lime, long bean, lahpet, and ngapi these salads are popular in Burmese cuisine.

Malaysian cuisine:
Malaysian cuisine has influenced the Indian, Chinese, and Malay. Malaysian cuisine is somewhat similar to Indonesian foods. Many of the same dishes are shared between these two countries. Nasi lemak is one of the popular dishes based on rice steamed with coconut milk. Pandan leaves are used as a fresh herb it gives rich fragrance to the dish. Nasi lemak is referred to as a national dish of Malaysia.

Sri Lankan cuisine:
Sri Lankan cuisines are influenced by south Indian, Dutch and Indonesian cuisine. Most of the Sri Lankan dishes are vegetarian, rice and curry, this is the most common food in Sri Lanka. Kiribath is a traditional Sri Lankan dish basically made from rice.

Thai cuisine:
Thai cuisine includes lightly prepared dishes with strong aromatic ingredients and spicy edge. Thai cuisine has not only great flavor but also comes with various medicinal benefits. Thai foods are balanced with five flavors like sweet, sour, salty, bitter and spicy. Pad Thai is the national dish of Thailand. The dish is made with chewy vegetables, stir-fried rice, peanut, eggs and bean sprouts with other herbs.

Singapore cuisine:
Singapore cuisines are influenced by Chinese, Indian, Malay, Indonesian and western food culture. Hainanese chicken rice is one of the popular national dishes in Singapore. In Hainanese culture rice is cooked with chicken fat and served with boiled chicken and chili sauce. Another popular dish is Sambal Stingray, a Singaporean seafood dish.

ADVANTAGES OF ASIAN MEALS AND CUISINE

Asian meals come with various health benefits which are described as follows:

- **Consumption of soy:** Soybean products are used in Asian cuisine; the phytoestrogens, estrogenic and antioxidant properties of its flavones help to reduce the cholesterol, improve bone health and prevent against heart disease.
- **Consumption of cold water fish:** Eating halibut, mackerel, salmon and other cold water fish are good for your health because fish contains an omega-3 fatty acid. It is very helpful in preventing and managing heart disease.
- **Eat a variety of green vegetables and fruits:** Green vegetables and fruits are loaded with vitamins like vitamin A, Vitamin-C, folate and potassium and fiber. It will help you to reduce the risk of obesity, high blood pressure, mental decline, and heart disease.

CHICKEN RECIPES
1-Flavorful Tandoori Chicken

Preparation Time: 10 minutes
Cooking Time: 15 minutes
Serve: 4

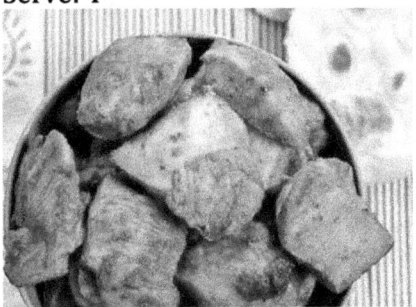

Ingredients:
- 1 lb chicken tenders, cut each in half
- 3/4 tsp garam masala
- ½ tsp turmeric
- ½ tsp chili powder
- ¼ cup fresh parsley, chopped
- 1 tbsp ginger garlic paste
- ¼ cup yogurt
- 1 tbsp olive oil
- ¾ tsp salt

Directions:
- Add all ingredients except oil into the large bowl and mix well and set aside for 30 minutes.
- Preheat the air fryer to 350 F/ 180 C for 5 minutes.
- Spray air fryer basket from inside with cooking spray.
- Place marinated chicken into the air fryer basket. Brush chicken with olive oil.
- Air fry at 350 F/ 180 C for 10 minutes.
- Turn chicken to another side and air fry for 5 minutes more.
- Serve and enjoy.

Nutritional Value (Amount per Serving):
- Calories 266
- Fat 12.5 g
- Carbohydrates 2.4 gs
- Sugar 1.1 g
- Protein 34.1 g
- Cholesterol 102 mg

2-Stir Fry Chicken

Preparation Time: 10 minutes
Cooking Time: 20 minutes
Serve: 4

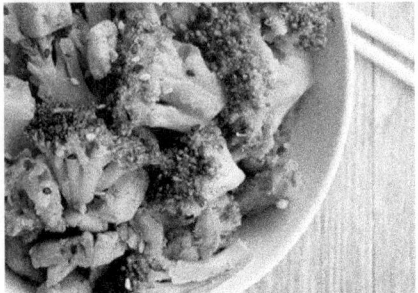

Ingredients:
- 1 lb chicken breast, skinless, boneless, and cut into chunks
- 1 ½ tsps white vinegar
- 1 tsp sesame oil
- 1 tbsp soy sauce
- ½ tbsp ginger, minced
- ½ tsp garlic powder
- 1 tbsp olive oil
- 1 small onion, sliced
- 1 cup broccoli florets
- Pepper
- Salt

Directions:
- In a large mixing bowl, mix together chicken, onion, and broccoli.
- In a small bowl, mix together olive oil, vinegar, sesame oil, soy sauce, ginger, and garlic powder and pour over chicken and stir well.
- Transfer chicken mixture to air fryer basket and air fry at 380 F/195 C for 15-20 minutes. Shake air fryer basket halfway through.
- Make sure chicken is cooked. If not then air fry for 4-5 minutes more.
- Season with pepper and salt.
- Serve and enjoy.

Nutritional Value (Amount per Serving):
- Calories 190
- Fat 7.6 g
- Carbohydrates 4.2 g
- Sugar 1.3 g
- Protein 25.2 g
- Cholesterol 73 mg

3-Spicy Chicken Wings

Preparation Time: 10 minutes
Cooking Time: 25 minutes
Serve: 4

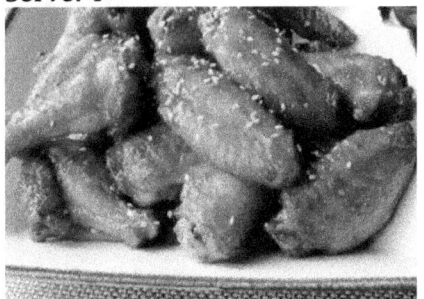

Ingredients:
- 1 lb chicken wings
- ¼ cup cornstarch
- Pepper
- Salt

For sauce:
- ½ fresh lime juice
- 1 tbsp olive oil
- 1 ¼ tbsps soy sauce
- 1 ½ tbsps sriracha sauce
- 3 tbsp honey

Directions:
- Preheat the air fryer to 375 F/ 190 C.
- In a large bowl, add chicken wings, cornstarch, pepper, and salt and toss until chicken wings are well coated.
- Spray air fryer basket from inside with cooking spray.
- Place chicken wings in the air fryer basket and air fry for 25 minutes.
- Turn chicken wings after every 5 minutes.
- Meanwhile, add all sauce ingredients into a small pan and bring to boil over low heat.
- Once wings are cooked then transfer them in mixing bowl. Pour sauce over chicken wings and toss well.
- Serve and enjoy.

Nutritional Value (Amount per Serving):
- Calories 365
- Fat 15.7 g
- Carbohydrates 21.5 g
- Sugar 13.5 g
- Protein 33.2 g
- Cholesterol 105 mg

4-Delicious Chicken Thighs

Preparation Time: 10 minutes
Cooking Time: 25 minutes
Serve: 6

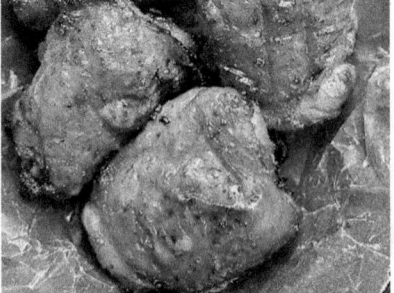

Ingredients:
- 6 chicken thighs, boneless
- ¾ tbsp onion powder
- ½ tbsp garlic powder
- 3 tbsps honey
- 2 tbsps lemon juice
- 1 tbsp Worcestershire sauce
- 3 tbsps soy sauce
- 1 tbsp sesame oil
- 2 tbsps olive oil
- ½ tsp kosher salt

Directions:
- Add all ingredients into the large bowl and mix until chicken is well coated.
- Spray air fryer basket from inside with cooking spray.
- Place chicken into the air fryer basket and air fry at 400 F/ 200 C for 15 minutes.
- Turn chicken to other side and air fry for 10 minutes more.
- Serve and enjoy.

Nutritional Value (Amount per Serving):
- Calories 383
- Fat 17.8 g
- Carbohydrates 11.1 g
- Sugar 9.9 g
- Protein 43 g
- Cholesterol 130 mg

5-Crispy Chicken Wings

Preparation Time: 10 minutes
Cooking Time: 34 minutes
Serve: 4

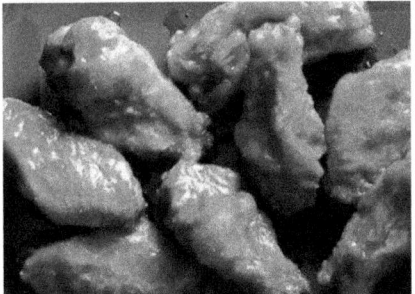

Ingredients:
- 2 lbs chicken wings
- ½ tsp onion powder
- 1 tsp garlic powder
- ½ cup cornstarch
- ½ tsp salt

For sauce:
- ½ tsp garlic, minced
- ½ tsp ginger, minced
- 1 tbsp soy sauce
- 1 ½ tbsps brown sugar
- 3 ½ tbsps honey
- 1 ½ tbsps chili paste
- ½ tsp salt

Directions:
- Add chicken wings in a large bowl and season with onion powder, garlic powder, and salt.
- Add cornstarch and toss until chicken wings are well coated.
- Place chicken wings in air fryer basket and air fry at 390 F/ 198 C for 30 minutes. Turn chicken after every 10 minutes.
- Meanwhile, add all sauce ingredients in a small pan and bring to boil and simmer over low heat for 3-4 minutes. Remove from heat and set aside.
- Transfer air fried chicken wings in a large bowl. Pour sauce over chicken wings and toss well.
- Serve and enjoy.

Nutritional Value (Amount per Serving):
- Calories 570
- Fat 17.8 g
- Carbohydrates 32.3 g
- Sugar 15.9 g
- Protein 66.5 g
- Cholesterol 204 mg

6-BBQ Chicken Wings

Preparation Time: 10 minutes
Cooking Time: 28 minutes
Serve: 2

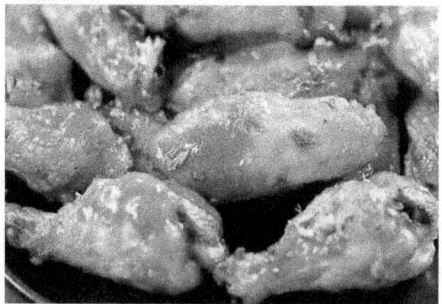

Ingredients:
- 6 chicken wings
- ½ tsp garlic powder
- ¼ tsp ginger powder
- 2 tsp soy sauce
- 4 tbsp honey BBQ sauce

Directions:
- Preheat the air fryer to 360 F/ 180 C.
- Place chicken wings in air fryer basket and air fry for 25-28 minutes. Shake basket after every 10 minutes.
- Meanwhile, in a bowl, mix together honey BBQ sauce, garlic powder, ginger powder, and soy sauce.
- Add air fried chicken wings in a sauce bowl and toss well to coat.
- Serve and enjoy.

Nutritional Value (Amount per Serving):
- Calories 422
- Fat 19.9 g
- Carbohydrates 29.1 g
- Sugar 22.3 g
- Protein 27.9 g
- Cholesterol 86 mg

7-Lemon Honey Chicken

Preparation Time: 10 minutes
Cooking Time: 15 minutes
Serve: 4

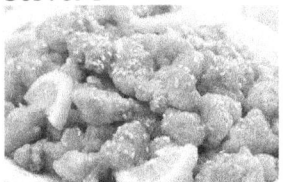

Ingredients:
- 1 egg, lightly beaten
- 1 lb chicken breast, skinless, boneless, and cut into chunks
- 1/3 cup breadcrumbs
- ½ cup cornstarch
- ¼ tsp pepper
- ¾ tsp salt

For sauce:
- 3 tbsps water
- 2 tbsps cornstarch
- ¼ tsp ginger, grated
- 1 tsp garlic powder
- 1 tsp sesame oil
- ½ tbsp lemon zest
- 2 ½ tbsps fresh lemon juice
- 2 tbsps white vinegar
- ¼ cup honey
- 1/3 cup soy sauce

Directions:
- Add all sauce ingredients in a saucepan and mix well. Take out 3 tablespoons of sauce mixture from saucepan and add in the large bowl. Set aside saucepan.
- Add egg in large bowl and mix well with 3 tablespoons of sauce.
- Add chicken in a bowl and mix well.
- In a large zip-lock bag, combine breadcrumbs, cornstarch, pepper, and salt. Add chicken and shake well to coat.
- Preheat the air fryer to 400 F/ 200 C for 8 minutes.
- Place chicken in air fryer basket and air fry for 8 minutes. Shake basket halfway through.
- Meanwhile for the sauce: Heat saucepan with sauce over medium-high heat. Stir constantly once the sauce is thickened then turn off the heat.
- Add air fried chicken in sauce and toss well to coat.
- Serve and enjoy.

Nutritional Value (Amount per Serving):
- Calories 350
- Fat 5.7 g
- Carbohydrates 45 g
- Sugar 18.8 g
- Protein 28.3 g
- Cholesterol 114 mg

8-Korean Chicken Wings

Preparation Time: 10 minutes
Cooking Time: 25 minutes
Serve: 4

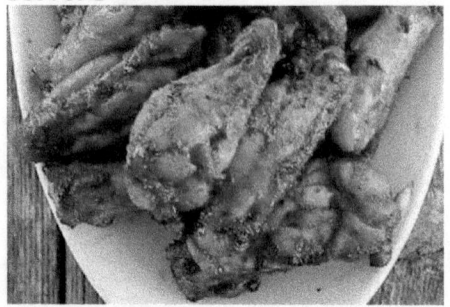

Ingredients:
- 2 lbs chicken wings
- ½ tsp pepper
- 1 tsp salt

For sauce:
- 2 tbsps sugar
- 1 tbsp garlic, minced
- 1 tbsp ginger, minced
- 1 tbsp sesame oil
- 1 tsp honey
- 1 tbsp mayonnaise
- 2 tbsps gochujang

Directions:
- Preheat the air fryer to 400 F/ 200 C.
- Season chicken wings with pepper and salt.
- Add chicken wings into the air fryer basket and air fry for 20 minutes. Turn halfway through.
- Meanwhile, in a bowl, mix together all sauce ingredients.
- Add air fried chicken wings to the sauce bowl and toss well.
- Return chicken wings to the air fryer basket and air fry for 5 minutes more.
- Serve and enjoy.

Nutritional Value (Amount per Serving):
- Calories 532
- Fat 21.5 g
- Carbohydrates 14.6 g
- Sugar 12.3 g
- Protein 66.4 g
- Cholesterol 203 mg

9-Tangy Chicken

Preparation Time: 10 minutes
Cooking Time: 15 minutes
Serve: 4

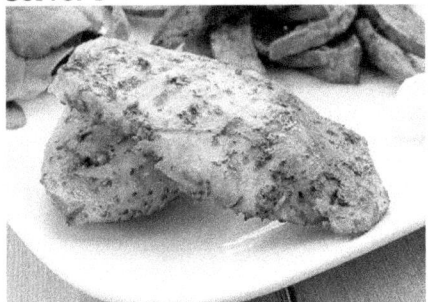

Ingredients:
- 4 chicken breast, skinless
- 2 tbsps Dijon mustard
- 3 tbsps olive oil
- 2 ½ tbsps soy sauce
- ¼ cup brown sugar
- ¼ cup balsamic vinegar

Directions:
- Add all ingredients except chicken in a bowl and mix well.
- Add chicken and mix until chicken is well coated and let marinate for 30 minutes.
- Place marinated chicken in air fryer basket and air fry at 380 F/ 193 C for 15 minutes.
- Serve and enjoy.

Nutritional Value (Amount per Serving):
- Calories 252
- Fat 13.3 g
- Carbohydrates 10.2 g
- Sugar 9.1 g
- Protein 22.2 g
- Cholesterol 64 mg

10-Sriracha Chicken Wings

Preparation Time: 10 minutes
Cooking Time: 33 minutes
Serve: 2

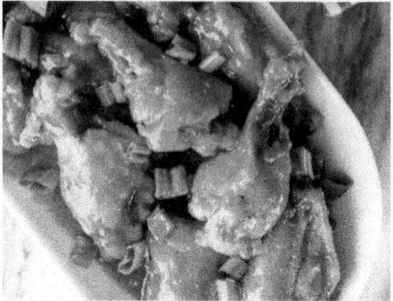

Ingredients:
- 1 lb chicken wings
- ½ fresh lime juice
- 1 tbsp butter
- 2 tbsps soy sauce
- 2 tbsps sriracha sauce
- 4 tbsps honey
- 2 tbsps green onion, chopped

Directions:
- Preheat the air fryer to 360 F/ 182 C.
- Add chicken wings to the air fryer basket and air fry for 30 minutes. Turn chicken after every 10 minutes.
- Meanwhile, add all remaining ingredients except green onion to a small pan and bring to boil for 3 minutes.
- Once chicken wings are cooked then toss with sauce until well coated.
- Garnish with green onion and serve.

Nutritional Value (Amount per Serving):
- Calories 361
- Fat 16.3 g
- Carbohydrates 19.1 g
- Sugar 18.1 g
- Protein 33.5 g
- Cholesterol 114 mg

MEAT RECIPES
11-Simple Air Fried Pork Chunks

Preparation Time: 10 minutes
Cooking Time: 12 minutes
Serve: 4

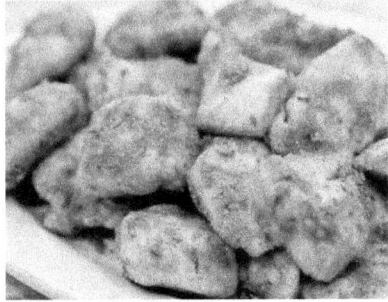

Ingredients:
- 2 eggs
- 2 lbs pork, cut into chunks
- 1 cup cornstarch
- ¼ tsp pepper
- ½ tsp sea salt

Directions:
- In a large bowl, mix together cornstarch, pepper, and salt.
- In another bowl, beat the eggs.
- Coat pork chunks with cornstarch mixture and dip each chunk into the egg mixture then again coat with cornstarch mixture.
- Spray air fryer basket from inside with cooking spray.
- Place pork chunks into the air fryer basket and air fry at 340 F/ 171 C for 10-12 minutes.
- Serve and enjoy.

Nutritional Value (Amount per Serving):
- Calories 478
- Fat 10.2 g
- Carbohydrates 29.5 g
- Sugar 0.2 g
- Protein 62.2 g
- Cholesterol 247 mg

12-Chinese Pork Roast

Preparation Time: 10 minutes
Cooking Time: 16 minutes
Serve: 4

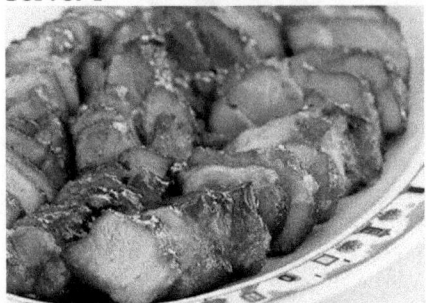

Ingredients:
- 1 lb pork shoulder, cut into slices
- ½ tsp Chinese five spice
- 1 ½ tsps ginger, minced
- 1 ½ tsps garlic, minced
- ½ tbsp hoisin sauce
- 1 tbsp rice wine
- 1 tbsp sugar
- 1 ½ tbsps soy sauce
- 3 tbsps honey

Directions:
- Add all ingredients except pork into the microwave-safe bowl and mix well.
- Add pork slices in a large bowl. Pour half the sauce over the pork slices and mix well and let marinate for half hour.
- Place marinated pork slices in air fryer basket and air fry at 390 F/ 198 C for 15 minutes. Turn meat halfway through.
- Meanwhile, microwave half the sauce for 40 seconds. Stir every 10 seconds.
- Once meat is cooked then brush with sauce and serve.

Nutritional Value (Amount per Serving):
- Calories 408
- Fat 24.4 g
- Carbohydrates 19.9 g
- Sugar 17.6 g
- Protein 27 g
- Cholesterol 102 mg

13-Spicy Korean Pork

Preparation Time: 10 minutes
Cooking Time: 15 minutes
Serve: 4

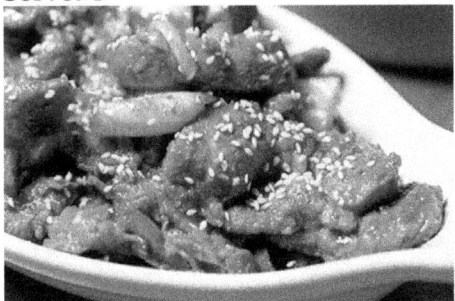

Ingredients:
- 1 lb pork shoulder, boneless and cut into slices
- 3 tbsps green onions, sliced
- ½ tbsp sesame seeds
- 2 tbsps chili paste
- 1 tsp sugar
- 1 tbsp sesame oil
- 1 tbsp rice wine
- 1 tbsp soy sauce
- 1 ½ tbsp ginger garlic paste
- 1 onion, sliced

Directions:
- In a large bowl, mix together pork, sugar, sesame oil, rice wine, soy sauce, ginger garlic paste, chili paste, and onion and let marinate for 30 minutes.
- Place marinated pork slices into the air fryer basket and air fry at 400 F/ 200 C for 15 minutes. Turn halfway through.
- Garnish with sesame seeds and green onion.
- Serve and enjoy.

Nutritional Value (Amount per Serving):
- Calories 427
- Fat 29.9 g
- Carbohydrates 10.3 g
- Sugar 5.3 g
- Protein 28.1 g
- Cholesterol 105 mg

14-Tasty BBQ Beef

Preparation Time: 10 minutes
Cooking Time: 20 minutes
Serve: 4

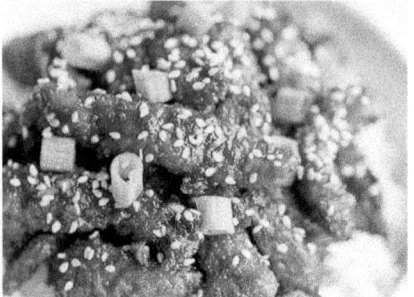

Ingredients:
- 1 lb flank steak, sliced
- ¼ cup cornstarch

For sauce:
- 1 tbsp water
- 1 tbsp cornstarch
- 1 tsp sesame seeds
- ½ tsp ginger powder
- 1 tbsp chili paste
- 1 garlic clove, minced
- 2 tbsps white vinegar
- ½ cup of soy sauce
- 6 tbsps brown sugar

Directions:
- Add sliced steak and cornstarch in a bowl and toss well to coat.
- Spray air fryer basket from inside with cooking spray.
- Place steak slices into the air fryer basket and air fry at 390 F/ 198 C for 10 minutes. Turn steak slices to other side and air fry for 10 minutes more.
- Meanwhile, add all sauce ingredients except water and cornstarch to a saucepan and bring to boil.
- Turn heat to low and whisk in water and cornstarch.
- Transfer air fried steak slices to the large mixing bowl and pour sauce over steak. Toss well.
- Serve and enjoy.

Nutritional Value (Amount per Serving):
- Calories 347
- Fat 10.4 g
- Carbohydrates 27 g
- Sugar 14.7 g
- Protein 34.1 g
- Cholesterol 64 mg

15-Crispy Pork Chops

Preparation Time: 10 minutes
Cooking Time: 13 minutes
Serve: 4

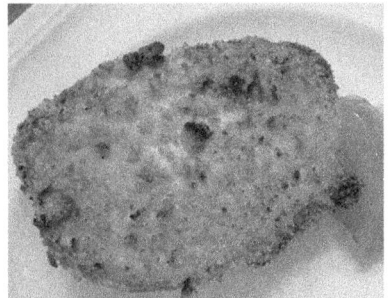

Ingredients:
- 6 pork chops, boneless
- 1 ½ cup seasoned breadcrumbs
- 2 egg, lightly beaten
- ¼ cup flour
- ¼ tsp pepper
- ¼ tsp salt

Directions:
- Add eggs, breadcrumbs, and flour in three separate shallow bowls.
- Season pork chops with pepper and salt.
- Coat pork chops with flour then dip in eggs and coat with breadcrumbs.
- Place pork chops in air fryer basket and air fry at 360 F/ 182 C for 8 minutes. Turn pork chops to other side and air fry for 5 minutes more.
- Serve and enjoy.

Nutritional Value (Amount per Serving):
- Calories 609
- Fat 37.4 g
- Carbohydrates 31.7 g
- Sugar 0.2 g
- Protein 35.1 g
- Cholesterol 185 mg

16-Ginger Garlic Beef

Preparation Time: 10 minutes
Cooking Time: 25 minutes
Serve: 4

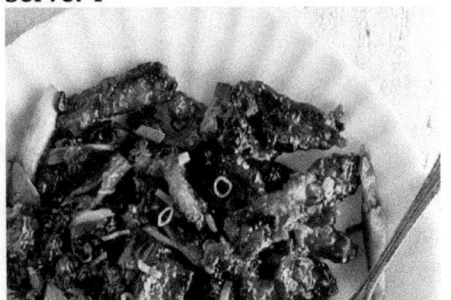

Ingredients:
- 1 lb flank steak, sliced
- ¼ cup cornstarch

For sauce:
- ½ cup brown sugar
- ½ cup of water
- ½ cup of soy sauce
- 1 tbsp garlic, minced
- ½ tsp ginger, minced
- 2 tbsps canola oil

Directions:
- Add sliced steak and cornstarch in a large bowl and toss well to coat.
- Place sliced steak into the air fryer basket and air fry at 390 F/ 198 C for 10 minutes.
- Turn sliced steak pieces to other side and air fry for 10 minutes more.
- Meanwhile, add all sauce ingredients in a saucepan and heat over medium-high heat. Cook sauce until begins to low boil. Remove from heat.
- Once steak is cooked then add in sauce mixture and let it soak for 5 minutes.
- Remove steak from the sauce and serve.

Nutritional Value (Amount per Serving):
- Calories 402
- Fat 16.5 g
- Carbohydrates 28.4 g
- Sugar 18.2 g
- Protein 33.7 g
- Cholesterol 62 mg

17-Spicy Lamb

Preparation Time: 10 minutes
Cooking Time: 10 minutes
Serve: 4

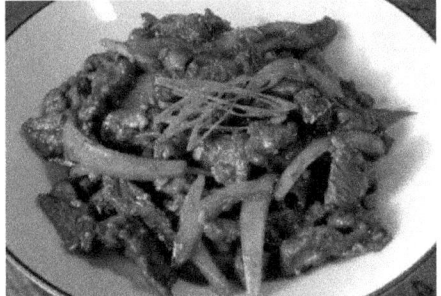

Ingredients:
- 1 lb lamb, cut into ½ inch pieces
- ¼ tsp sugar
- 1 ½ red chili peppers, chopped
- 1 tbsp garlic, minced
- ¾ tbsp soy sauce
- 2 tbsps canola oil
- ½ tsp cayenne
- ½ tbsp cumin powder
- 2 tbsps green onion, chopped
- 1 tsp salt

Directions:
- In a large bowl, mix together lamb, cumin powder, cayenne, sugar, red chili peppers, garlic, soy sauce, oil, and salt.
- Place marinated lamb pieces into the air fryer basket and air fry at 360 F/ 182 C for 10 minutes.
- Garnish with green onion and serve.

Nutritional Value (Amount per Serving):
- Calories 286
- Fat 15.7 g
- Carbohydrates 2.3 g
- Sugar 0.5 g
- Protein 32.5 g
- Cholesterol 102 mg

18-Beef Kabab

Preparation Time: 10 minutes
Cooking Time: 10 minutes
Serve: 4

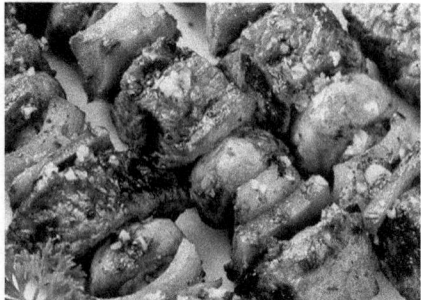

Ingredients:
- 1 lb beef, cut into chunks
- ½ onion, cut into 1-inch pieces
- 1 bell pepper, cut into 1-inch pieces
- 2 tbsps soy sauce
- 1/3 cup sour cream

Directions:
- In a bowl, mix together soy sauce and sour cream.
- Add beef chunks into the bowl and mix well and let marinate for 30 minutes.
- Soak wooden skewers in water for 15 minutes.
- Thread marinated beef chunks, bell peppers, and onions onto skewers.
- Place prepared skewers in air fryer basket and air fry at 400 F/ 200 C for 10 minutes. Turn halfway through.
- Serve and enjoy.

Nutritional Value (Amount per Serving):
- Calories 271
- Fat 11.2 g
- Carbohydrates 5 g
- Sugar 2.3 g
- Protein 36 g
- Cholesterol 110 mg

19-Crispy Grilled Pork

Preparation Time: 10 minutes
Cooking Time: 10 minutes
Serve: 4

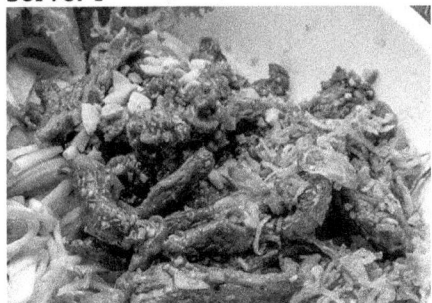

Ingredients:
- 1 lb pork shoulder, sliced
- 1 tbsp lemongrass, minced
- ½ tbsp fish sauce
- 1 ½ tsp soy sauce
- 1 tbsp garlic, minced
- 2 tbsps sugar
- 2 tbsps canola oil
- 3 tbsps onion, minced
- 2 tbsps fresh parsley, chopped

Directions:
- In a medium bowl, whisk together onions, lemongrass, fish sauce, garlic, oil, soy sauce, and sugar.
- Add sliced pork into the bowl and mix well and let marinate for 30 minutes.
- Place marinated pork slices into the air fryer basket and air fry at 400 F/ 200 C for 10 minutes. Turn halfway through.
- Garnish with fresh parsley and serve.

Nutritional Value (Amount per Serving):
- Calories 425
- Fat 31.3 g
- Carbohydrates 8 g
- Sugar 6.5 g
- Protein 26.9 g
- Cholesterol 102 mg

20-Flavorful Lamb Steak

Preparation Time: 10 minutes
Cooking Time: 15 minutes
Serve: 4

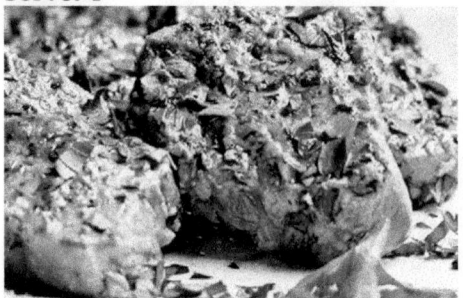

Ingredients:
- 1 lb lamb chops, boneless
- 1 tsp cayenne
- ½ tsp cardamom powder
- ¼ tsp ground fennel
- ½ tsp garam masala
- 3 garlic cloves
- 1 tbsp ginger, sliced
- ½ onion, sliced
- 1 tsp salt

Directions:
- Add all ingredients except meat into the blender and blend all ingredients for 3-4 minutes.
- Add meat into the large bowl and pour blended mixture over meat and mix well. Marinate meat for 30 minutes.
- Place marinated meat into the air fryer basket and air fry at 330 F/ 165 C for 15 minutes. Turn meat halfway through.
- Serve and enjoy.

Nutritional Value (Amount per Serving):
- Calories 227
- Fat 8.5 g
- Carbohydrates 3.5 g
- Sugar 0.7 g
- Protein 32.4 g
- Cholesterol 102 mg

FISH & SEAFOOD RECIPES
21-Garlic Lemon Shrimp

Preparation Time: 10 minutes
Cooking Time: 6 minutes
Serve: 4

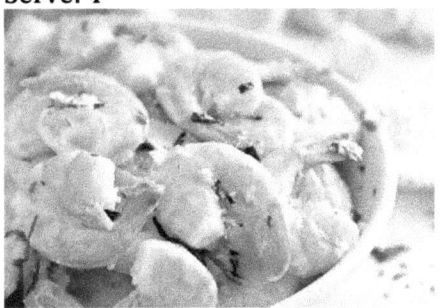

Ingredients:
- 1 lb shrimp, deveined and peeled
- 1 tbsp fresh lemon juice
- 3 garlic cloves, minced
- ¼ tsp cayenne pepper
- 1 tbsp honey
- 2 tbsps soy sauce
- 2 tbsps olive oil
- ¼ tsp pepper
- ¼ tsp kosher salt

Directions:
- Add shrimp into the large bowl.
- Add remaining ingredients to the shrimp bowl and mix well and let marinate for 15 minutes.
- Place marinated shrimp into the air fryer basket and air fry at 410 F/ 210 C for 6 minutes.
- Serve and enjoy.

Nutritional Value (Amount per Serving):
- Calories 220
- Fat 9 g
- Carbohydrates 7.6 g
- Sugar 4.6 g
- Protein 26.5 g
- Cholesterol 239 mg

22-Salmon Patties

Preparation Time: 10 minutes
Cooking Time: 8 minutes
Serve: 6

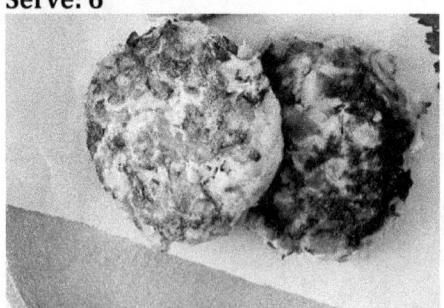

Ingredients:
- 14 oz can salmon, bone removed and drained
- 2 eggs, lightly beaten
- ½ lime zest
- 1 tbsps brown sugar
- 2 tbsps red curry paste
- ½ cup breadcrumbs
- ¼ tsp salt

Directions:
- Add all ingredients into the bowl and mix until well combined.
- Make round patties from mixture and place in air fryer basket.
- Spray patties with cooking spray.
- Air fry patties at 360 F/ 182 C for 4 minutes then turns to other side and air fry for 4 minutes more.
- Serve and enjoy.

Nutritional Value (Amount per Serving):
- Calories 174
- Fat 7.4 g
- Carbohydrates 9.1 g
- Sugar 2.1 g
- Protein 16.1 g
- Cholesterol 91 mg

23-Shrimp with Sauce

Preparation Time: 10 minutes
Cooking Time: 9 minutes
Serve: 4

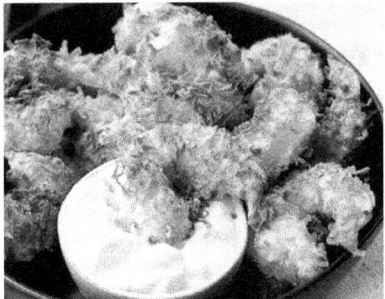

Ingredients:
- 1 egg
- 1 tbsp fresh parsley, chopped
- ½ lb shrimp, peeled and deveined
- ½ cup breadcrumbs
- 2 tbsps cornstarch
- ¼ tsp salt

For sauce:
- 1 tsp sesame oil
- ½ tsp paprika
- ½ tbsp brown sugar
- 1 tbsp white vinegar
- ½ tbsp chili sauce
- 1 garlic clove, minced
- 1 tbsp butter, melted
- ½ cup mayonnaise

Directions:
- Add all sauce ingredients in a small bowl and mix well and set aside.
- Add eggs, breadcrumbs, and cornstarch in three separate shallow dishes.
- Coat shrimp with cornstarch then dip in egg mixture and finally coat with breadcrumbs.
- Place parchment paper piece in air fryer basket.
- Place shrimp on parchment paper and air fry at 350 F/ 176 C for 4 minutes. Turn shrimp to other side and air fry for 4-5 minutes more.
- Garnish with parsley and serve with sauce.

Nutritional Value (Amount per Serving):
- Calories 309
- Fat 16.6 g
- Carbohydrates 23 g
- Sugar 4 g
- Protein 16.5 g
- Cholesterol 176 mg

24-Honey Soy Salmon

Preparation Time: 10 minutes
Cooking Time: 12 minutes
Serve: 2

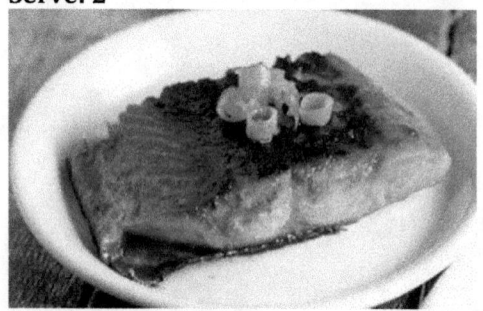

Ingredients:
- 2 salmon fillets, skin on
- ¾ tbsp soy sauce
- 3 tbsps sriracha
- 6 tbsps honey

Directions:
- In a bowl, mix together soy sauce, sriracha, and honey.
- Add salmon fillets to the bowl and coat well with the sauce and let marinate for 30 minutes.
- Spray air fryer basket from inside with cooking spray.
- Place marinated salmon in air fryer basket and air fry at 400 F/ 200 C for 12 minutes.
- Serve and enjoy.

Nutritional Value (Amount per Serving):
- Calories 453
- Fat 11 g
- Carbohydrates 56.9 g
- Sugar 51.8 g
- Protein 35.1 g
- Cholesterol 78 mg

25-Tasty Asian Shrimp

Preparation Time: 10 minutes
Cooking Time: 10 minutes
Serve: 4

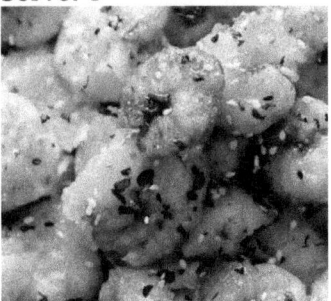

Ingredients:
- 1 lb shrimp, peeled and deveined
- ¼ tsp ginger, minced
- 2 garlic cloves, minced
- 2 ½ tbsps soy sauce
- 2 ½ tbsps chili sauce
- 1 tbsp cornstarch

Directions:
- Spray air fryer basket from inside with cooking spray.
- Coat shrimp with cornstarch and place into the air fryer basket.
- Air fry shrimp at 350 F/ 176 C for 5 minutes. Turn shrimp to other side and spray with cooking spray and air fry for 5 minutes more.
- Meanwhile, for the sauce in a bowl, mix together remaining ingredients.
- Add air fried shrimp in a sauce bowl and toss well.
- Serve and enjoy.

Nutritional Value (Amount per Serving):
- Calories 151
- Fat 2 g
- Carbohydrates 5.1 g
- Sugar 0.3 g
- Protein 26.6 g
- Cholesterol 239 mg

26-Healthy Salmon Patties

Preparation Time: 10 minutes
Cooking Time: 7 minutes
Serve: 2

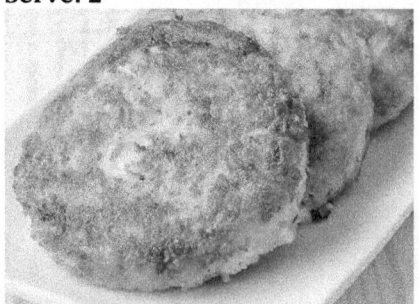

Ingredients:
- 1 egg, lightly beaten
- 8 oz fresh salmon fillet, mince
- ½ tsp garlic powder
- 2 tbsps fresh parsley, chopped
- 1/8 tsp salt

Directions:
- Preheat the air fryer to 390 F/ 198 C for 5 minutes.
- Add all ingredients into the bowl and mix well to combine.
- Make patties from mixture and place in air fryer basket.
- Air fry patties in preheated air fryer for 7 minutes.
- Serve and enjoy.

Nutritional Value (Amount per Serving):
- Calories 184
- Fat 9.2 g
- Carbohydrates 0.7 g
- Sugar 0.3 g
- Protein 24.9 g
- Cholesterol 132 mg

27-Sriracha Salmon

Preparation Time: 10 minutes
Cooking Time: 14 minutes
Serve: 2

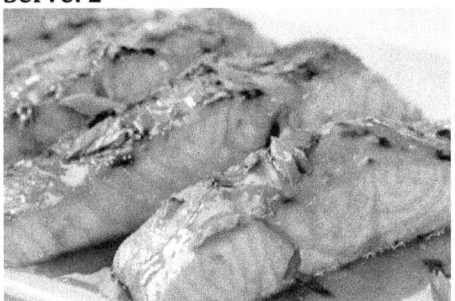

Ingredients:
- 2 salmon fillets
- ½ tbsp soy sauce
- 1 ½ tbsp sriracha
- 1 ½ tbsp white vinegar
- 1/3 cup ketchup
- 1/3 cup bourbon
- 6 tbsps brown sugar

Directions:
- In a saucepan, combine together brown sugar, soy sauce, sriracha, vinegar, ketchup, and bourbon. Bring to boil.
- Turn heat to low and simmer for 8 minutes.
- Brush salmon fillet with sauce and place in air fryer basket.
- Air fry salmon at 400 F/ 200 C for 14 minutes.
- Serve with sauce and enjoy.

Nutritional Value (Amount per Serving):
- Calories 478
- Fat 11.1 g
- Carbohydrates 39.2 g
- Sugar 35.4 g
- Protein 35.5 g
- Cholesterol 78 mg

28-Ginger Garlic Shrimp

Preparation Time: 10 minutes
Cooking Time: 10 minutes
Serve: 4

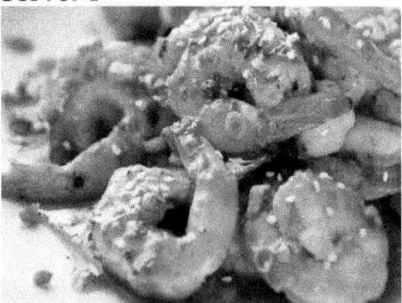

Ingredients:
- 1 lb shrimp, peeled and deveined
- 1/8 tsp ginger, minced
- 2 garlic cloves, minced
- 2 tbsps soy sauce
- 1 tsp sesame seeds
- 1 tbsp green onion, sliced
- 2 tbsps Thai chili sauce
- 1 tbsp cornstarch

Directions:
- Spray air fryer basket with cooking spray.
- Toss shrimp with cornstarch and place into the air fryer basket.
- Air fry shrimp at 350 F/ 176 C for 5 minutes. Shake basket well and cook for 5 minutes more.
- Meanwhile, in a bowl, mix together soy sauce, ginger, garlic, and chili sauce.
- Add shrimp to the bowl and mix well.
- Sprinkle with green onions and sesame seeds.
- Serve and enjoy.

Nutritional Value (Amount per Serving):
- Calories 164
- Fat 2.3 g
- Carbohydrates 7.5 g
- Sugar 2.2 g
- Protein 26.6 g
- Cholesterol 239 mg

29-Lemon Chili Shrimp

Preparation Time: 10 minutes
Cooking Time: 7 minutes
Serve: 4

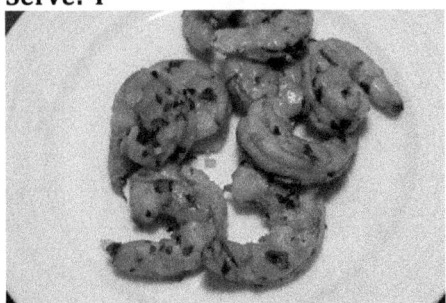

Ingredients:
- 1 lb shrimp, peeled and deveined
- 1 tbsp canola oil
- 1 lemon, sliced
- 1 red chili, sliced
- 1/2 tsp garlic powder
- Pepper
- Salt

Directions:
- Preheat the air fryer to 400 F/ 200 C.
- Spray air fryer basket with cooking spray.
- Add all ingredients into the mixing bowl and toss well.
- Transfer shrimp mixture into the air fryer basket and air fry for 5 minutes.
- Shake basket well and cook for 2 minutes more.
- Serve and enjoy.

Nutritional Value (Amount per Serving):
- Calories 167
- Fat 5.4 g
- Carbohydrates 2 g
- Sugar 0.1 g
- Protein 25.9 g
- Cholesterol 239 mg

30-Crispy Coconut Shrimp

Preparation Time: 10 minutes
Cooking Time: 5 minutes
Serve: 4

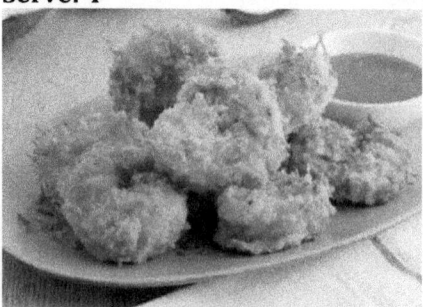

Ingredients:
- 16 oz shrimp, peeled
- 2 egg whites
- 1/4 tsp cayenne pepper
- 1/2 cup shredded coconut
- 1/2 cup breadcrumbs
- 1/2 tsp salt

Directions:
- Preheat the air fryer at 400 F/ 200 C.
- Spray air fryer basket with cooking spray.
- Whisk egg whites in a shallow dish.
- In a bowl, mix together shredded coconut, breadcrumbs, and cayenne pepper.
- Dip shrimp into the egg mixture then coat with coconut mixture and place into the air fryer basket.
- Air fry at 400 F/ 200 C for 5 minutes.
- Serve and enjoy.

Nutritional Value (Amount per Serving):
- Calories 232
- Fat 6 g
- Carbohydrates 13.1 g
- Sugar 1.6 g
- Protein 29.8 g
- Cholesterol 239 mg

SIDE DISHES

31-Sweet Potato Bites

Preparation Time: 10 minutes
Cooking Time: 15 minutes
Serve: 2

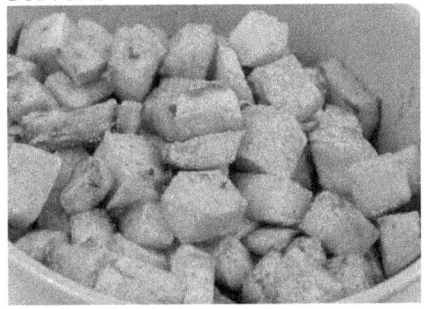

Ingredients:
- 2 sweet potato, diced into 1-inch cubes
- 1 tsp red chili flakes
- 1/2 cup fresh parsley, chopped
- 1 1/2 tsps cinnamon
- 2 tbsps canola oil
- 2 tbsps honey

Directions:
- Preheat air fryer at 350 F/ 176 C.
- Add all ingredients into the bowl and toss well.
- Place sweet potato mixture into the air fryer basket.
- Cook in preheated air fryer for 15 minutes.
- Serve and enjoy.

Nutritional Value (Amount per Serving):
- Calories 300
- Fat 14.3 g
- Carbohydrates 43.2 g
- Sugar 24.8 g
- Protein 2.9 g
- Cholesterol 0 mg

32-Crispy Cauliflower Florets

Preparation Time: 10 minutes
Cooking Time: 20 minutes
Serve: 2

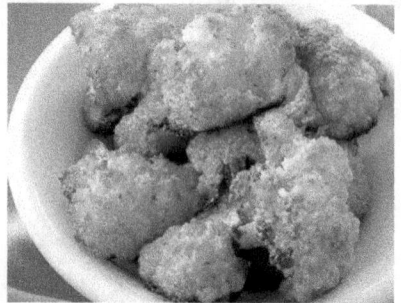

Ingredients:
- 2 cups cauliflower florets, boiled
- 1 egg, beaten
- 1 tbsp canola oil
- 1/4 cup flour
- 1/2 cup breadcrumbs
- 1/2 tsp garlic powder
- 1/2 tsp chili powder
- 1/2 tbsp mix herb
- 2 tbsps parmesan cheese, grated
- Salt

Directions:
- In a bowl, combine together breadcrumbs, garlic powder, chili powder, mix herb, salt, and cheese.
- Add oil in breadcrumbs mixture and mix well.
- Add flour in shallow dish and beaten egg in small bowl.
- Dip cauliflower floret in beaten egg then in flour and finally coat with breadcrumbs.
- Preheat the air fryer at 350 F/ 176 C.
- Place coated cauliflower florets in air fryer basket and air fry for 20 minutes. Shake basket halfway through.
- Serve and enjoy.

Nutritional Value (Amount per Serving):
- Calories 286
- Fat 11 g
- Carbohydrates 37.7 g
- Sugar 4.5 g
- Protein 10.2 g
- Cholesterol 82 mg

33-Banana Chips

Preparation Time: 10 minutes
Cooking Time: 15 minutes
Serve: 3

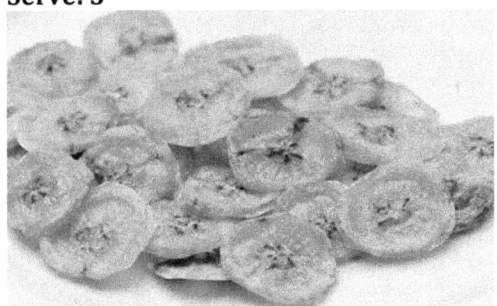

Ingredients:
- 2 large raw bananas, peel and sliced
- 1 tsp canola oil
- 1/4 tsp turmeric powder
- 1/2 tsp red chili powder
- 1 tsp salt

Directions:
- In a bowl add water, turmeric powder, and salt. Stir well.
- Add sliced bananas in bowl water soak for 10 minutes. Drain well and dry chips with a paper towel.
- Preheat the air fryer to 350 F/ 176 C.
- Add banana slices in mixing bowl and toss with oil, chili powder, and salt.
- Place banana slices in air fryer basket and air fry for 15 minutes. Shake basket halfway through.
- Serve and enjoy.

Nutritional Value (Amount per Serving):
- Calories 96
- Fat 2 g
- Carbohydrates 21.1 g
- Sugar 11.1 g
- Protein 1.1 g
- Cholesterol 0 mg

34-Broccoli with Pine Nuts

Preparation Time: 10 minutes
Cooking Time: 15 minutes
Serve: 6

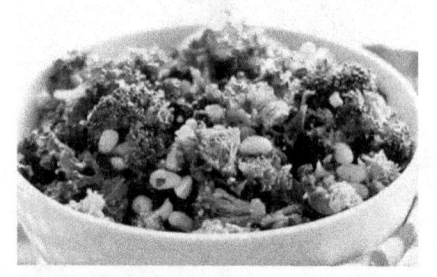

Ingredients:
- 1 lb broccoli florets
- 1 tbsp garlic, minced
- 1 1/2 tbsps canola oil
- 1 fresh lime juice
- 1/4 cup pine nuts
- 1 tsp rice vinegar
- 2 tsps sriracha
- 2 tbsps soy sauce
- Salt

Directions:
- In a bowl, toss together broccoli, oil, salt, and garlic.
- Add broccoli into the air fryer basket and air fry at 400 F/ 200 C for 15 minutes. Shake basket halfway through.
- Meanwhile, in a microwave safe bowl, mix together rice vinegar, sriracha, and soy sauce and microwave for 10 seconds.
- Transfer air fried broccoli into the large bowl.
- Pour vinegar mixture over the broccoli and toss well.
- Add lime juice and pine nuts and toss well.
- Serve and enjoy.

Nutritional Value (Amount per Serving):
- Calories 102
- Fat 7.6 g
- Carbohydrates 7 g
- Sugar 1.6 g
- Protein 3.3 g
- Cholesterol 0 mg

35-Garlic Cauliflower Florets

Preparation Time: 10 minutes
Cooking Time: 20 minutes
Serve: 4

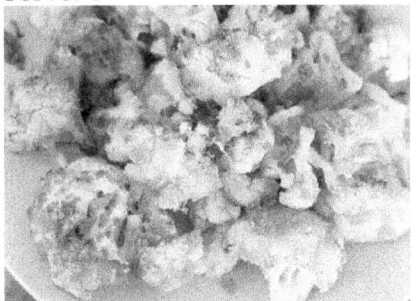

Ingredients:
- 5 cups cauliflower florets
- 6 garlic cloves, chopped
- 1/2 tsp cumin powder
- 4 tablespoons canola oil
- 1/2 tsp coriander powder
- 1/2 tsp salt

Directions:
- Add all ingredients into the large bowl and toss well.
- Add cauliflower florets into the air fryer basket and air fry at 400 F/ 200 C for 20 minutes. Shake basket halfway through.
- Serve and enjoy.

Nutritional Value (Amount per Serving):
- Calories 163
- Fat 14.2 g
- Carbohydrates 8.2 g
- Sugar 3.1 g
- Protein 2.8 g
- Cholesterol 0 mg

VEGETARIAN & TOFU RECIPES
36-Roasted Broccoli with Peanuts

Preparation Time: 10 minutes
Cooking Time: 20 minutes
Serve: 4

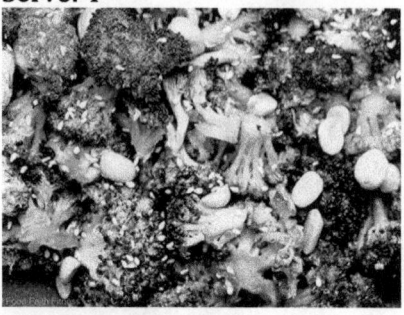

Ingredients:
- 1 lb broccoli, cut into florets
- 1/3 cup peanuts, roasted
- 1 tsp white vinegar
- 2 tsps sriracha
- 2 tsps honey
- 2 tbsps soy sauce
- 1 tbsp garlic, minced
- 1 ½ tbsps canola oil
- Salt

Directions:
- In a large mixing bowl, toss broccoli with garlic, oil, and salt.
- Add broccoli into the air fryer basket and air fry at 400 F/ 200 C for 15-20 minutes. Shake basket halfway through.
- Meanwhile, in a microwave-safe bowl, mix together honey, vinegar, sriracha, and soy sauce and microwave for 10-15 seconds.
- Transfer air fried broccoli to the large bowl. Add peanuts and honey mixture over broccoli and toss well.
- Serve and enjoy.

Nutritional Value (Amount per Serving):
- Calories 175
- Fat 11.6 g
- Carbohydrates 14.2 g
- Sugar 5.5 g
- Protein 7 g
- Cholesterol 0 mg

37-Garlic Brussels sprouts

Preparation Time: 10 minutes
Cooking Time: 8 minutes
Serve: 4

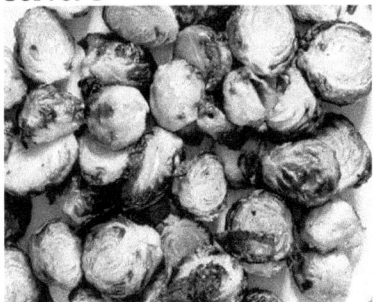

Ingredients:
- 1 lb Brussels sprouts, clean and trimmed
- 2 tsps canola oil
- 4 garlic cloves, minced
- 1 tsp dried parsley
- ¼ tsp salt

Directions:
- Add all ingredients into the large bowl and toss well.
- Pour Brussels sprouts mixture into the air fryer basket and air fry at 390 F/ 198 C for 8 minutes.
- Serve and enjoy.

Nutritional Value (Amount per Serving):
- Calories 74
- Fat 2.7 g
- Carbohydrates 11.3 g
- Sugar 2.5 g
- Protein 4.1 g
- Cholesterol 0 mg

38-Delicious Air Fried Tofu

Preparation Time: 10 minutes
Cooking Time: 20 minutes
Serve: 4

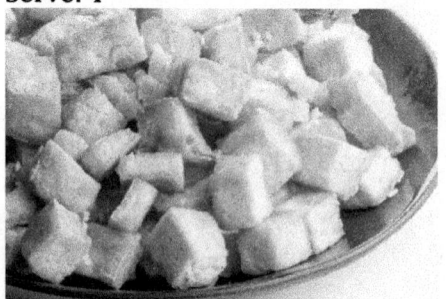

Ingredients:
- 1 block firm tofu, cut into 1-inch cubes
- 1 tbsp cornstarch
- 2 tsps sesame oil
- 1 tsp white vinegar
- 2 tbsps soy sauce

Directions:
- Add tofu, sesame oil, vinegar, and soy sauce in a large bowl and let it marinate for 15 minutes.
- Toss marinated tofu with cornstarch and place in air fryer basket.
- Air fry tofu at 370 F/ 187 C for 20 minutes. Shake basket halfway through.
- Serve and enjoy.

Nutritional Value (Amount per Serving):
- Calories 48
- Fat 3.2 g
- Carbohydrates 2.8 g
- Sugar 0.3 g
- Protein 2.4 g
- Cholesterol 0 mg

39-Lemon Garlic Broccoli Florets

Preparation Time: 10 minutes
Cooking Time: 13 minutes
Serve: 4

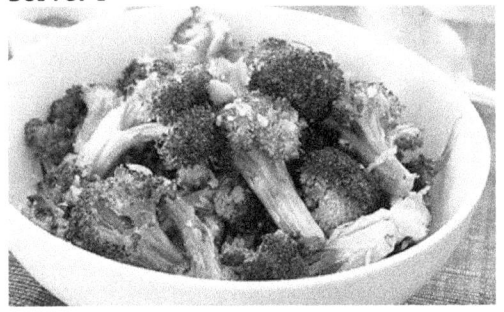

Ingredients:
- 1 lb broccoli, cut into florets
- 1 tbsp fresh lemon juice
- 3 garlic cloves, minced
- 1 tbsp olive oil
- 1 tbsp sesame seeds

Directions:
- Add all ingredients into the bowl and toss well.
- Add broccoli into the air fryer basket and air fry at 400 F/ 200 C for 13 minutes.
- Serve and enjoy.

Nutritional Value (Amount per Serving):
- Calories 86
- Fat 5 g
- Carbohydrates 8.9 g
- Sugar 2 g
- Protein 3.8 g
- Cholesterol 0 mg

40-Crispy Tofu

Preparation Time: 10 minutes
Cooking Time: 8 minutes
Serve: 4

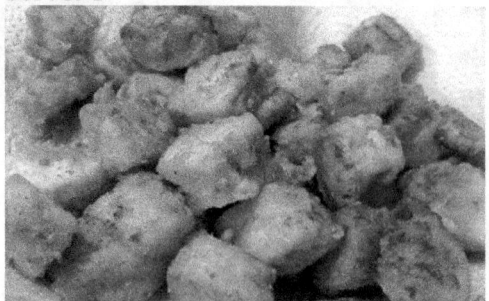

Ingredients:
- 15 oz firm tofu, drain and cut into cubes
- 3/4 cup cornstarch
- 1/4 cup cornmeal
- 1 tsp chili flakes
- Pepper
- Salt

Directions:
- In a bowl, mix together cornmeal, cornstarch, chili flakes, pepper, and salt.
- Add tofu cubes in cornmeal mixture and coat well.
- Preheat air fryer at 350 F/ 176 C.
- Spray air fryer basket with cooking spray.
- Place coated tofu in air fryer basket and air fry for 8 minutes. Shake basket halfway through.
- Serve with enjoy.

Nutritional Value (Amount per Serving):
- Calories 194
- Fat 4.7 g
- Carbohydrates 29.6 g
- Sugar 0.7 g
- Protein 9.4 g
- Cholesterol 0 mg

DESSERTS & SNACKS
41-Delicious Chinese Doughnuts

Preparation Time: 10 minutes
Cooking Time: 8 minutes
Serve: 8

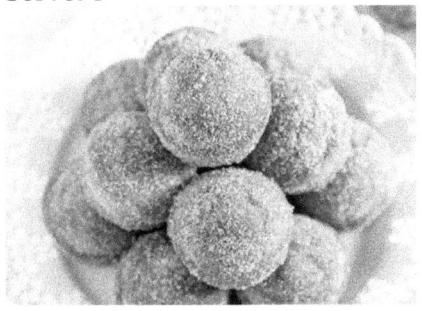

Ingredients:
- 2 cups all-purpose flour
- ¾ cup of coconut milk
- 6 tbsps coconut oil
- 1 tbsp baking powder
- 2 tsps sugar
- ½ tsp sea salt

Directions:
- Preheat the air fryer to 350 F/ 176 C.
- In a bowl, mix together flour, baking powder, sugar, and salt.
- Add coconut oil and mix well. Add coconut milk and mix until well combined.
- Knead dough for 3-4 minutes.
- Roll dough half inch thick and using cookie cutter cut doughnuts.
- Place doughnuts in cake pan and brush with oil. Place cake pan in air fryer basket and air fry doughnuts for 5 minutes. Turn doughnuts to other side and air fry for 3 minutes more.
- Serve and enjoy.

Nutritional Value (Amount per Serving):
- Calories 259
- Fat 15.9 g
- Carbohydrates 27 g
- Sugar 1.8 g
- Protein 3.8 g
- Cholesterol 0 mg

42-Sweet & Crisp Bananas

Preparation Time: 10 minutes
Cooking Time: 10 minutes
Serve: 4

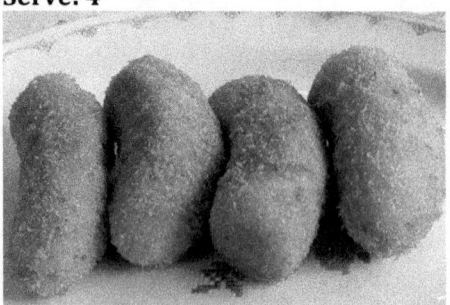

Ingredients:
- 4 ripe bananas, peeled and cut in half pieces
- 1 egg, beaten
- 1 1/2 tbsps Coconut Oil
- 1 tbsp almond meal
- 1 tbsp cashew, crushed
- 1/2 cup breadcrumbs
- 1/4 cup corn flour
- 1 1/2 tbsps cinnamon sugar

Directions:
- Heat coconut oil in a pan over medium heat and add breadcrumbs in the pan and stir for 3-4 minutes.
- Remove pan from heat and transfer breadcrumbs in a bowl.
- Add almond meal and crush cashew in breadcrumbs and mix well.
- Dip banana half in corn flour then in egg and finally coat with breadcrumbs.
- Place coated banana in air fryer basket. Sprinkle with Cinnamon Sugar.
- Air fry at 350 F/ 176 C for 10 minutes.
- Serve and enjoy.

Nutritional Value (Amount per Serving):
- Calories 282
- Fat 9 g
- Carbohydrates 46 g
- Sugar 15 g
- Protein 5 g
- Cholesterol 41 mg

43-Banana Muffins

Preparation Time: 10 minutes
Cooking Time: 10 minutes
Serve: 2

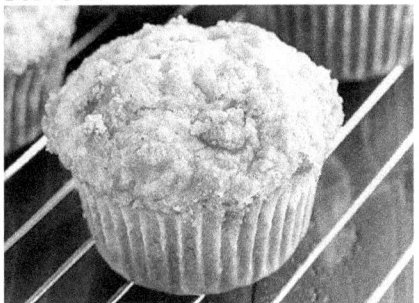

Ingredients:
- 1/4 cup banana, mashed
- 1/4 cup oats
- 1 tbsp walnuts, chopped
- 1/4 cup flour
- 1/2 tsp baking powder
- 1/4 cup powdered sugar
- 1/4 cup butter

Directions:
- Spray four muffin molds with cooking spray and set aside.
- In a bowl, mix together mashed banana, walnuts, sugar, and butter.
- In another bowl, mix together flour, baking powder, and oats.
- Add flour mixture to the banana mixture and mix well.
- Pour batter into the prepared muffin mold.
- Place in air fryer basket and cook at 320 F/ 160 C for 10 minutes.
- Remove muffins from air fryer and allow to cool completely.
- Serve and enjoy.

Nutritional Value (Amount per Serving):
- Calories 192
- Fat 12.3 g
- Carbohydrates 19.4 g
- Sugar 8.6 g
- Protein 1.9 g
- Cholesterol 31 mg

44-Easy Blueberry Muffins

Preparation Time: 10 minutes
Cooking Time: 14 minutes
Serve: 2

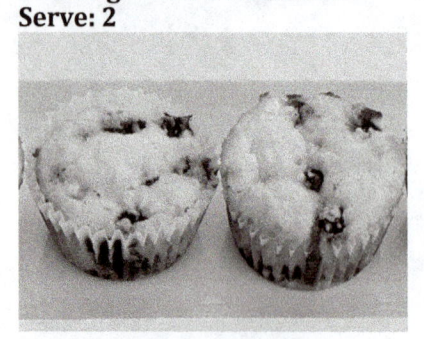

Ingredients:
- 1 egg
- 3/4 cup blueberries
- 2 tbsps sugar
- 1 tsp baking powder
- 2/3 cup flour
- 3 tbsps butter, melted
- 1/3 cup milk

Directions:
- Spray four silicone muffins cups with cooking spray and set aside.
- In a bowl, mix together all ingredients until well combined.
- Pour batter into the prepared muffins cups.
- Place muffin cups in air fryer basket and cook at 320 F/ 160 C for 14 minutes.
- Serve and enjoy.

Nutritional Value (Amount per Serving):
- Calories 435
- Fat 20.9 g
- Carbohydrates 55 g
- Sugar 19.5 g
- Protein 9 g
- Cholesterol 131 mg

45- Spicy Mix Nuts

Preparation Time: 5 minutes
Cooking Time: 4 minutes
Serve: 6

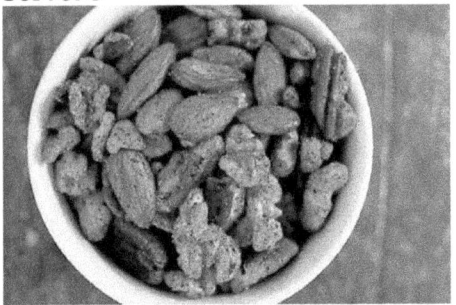

Ingredients:
- 2 cup mix nuts
- 1 tbsp butter, melted
- 1 tsp chili powder
- 1 tsp ground cumin
- 1 tsp pepper
- 1 tsp salt

Directions:
- Add all ingredients in a mixing bowl and toss until well coated.
- Preheat the air fryer at 350 F/ 176 C for 5 minutes.
- Add mix nuts in air fryer basket and air fry for 4 minutes. Shake basket halfway through.
- Serve and enjoy.

Nutritional Value (Amount per Serving):
- Calories 316
- Fat 29 g
- Carbohydrates 11.3 g
- Sugar 2.1 g
- Protein 7.6 g
- Cholesterol 5 mg

KETO ASIAN RECIPES
46-Healthy Air Fried Okra

Preparation Time: 10 minutes
Cooking Time: 15 minutes
Serve: 2

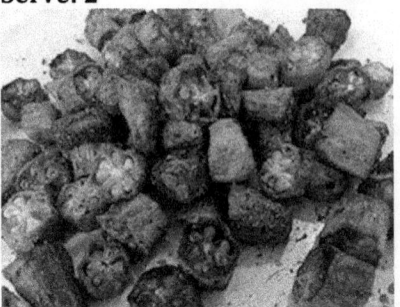

Ingredients:
- ½ lb okra, trimmed and sliced
- 1 tsp vegetable oil
- ¼ tsp chili powder
- ¼ tsp garlic powder
- 1/8 tsp pepper
- ¼ tsp salt

Directions:
- Preheat the air fryer to 350 F/ 176 C.
- Add all ingredients into the mixing bowl and toss well.
- Transfer okra into the air fryer basket and air fry for 10 minutes. Shake basket halfway through.
- Toss again and cook for 2 minutes more.
- Serve and enjoy.

Nutritional Value (Amount per Serving):
- Calories 68
- Fat 2.6 g
- Carbohydrates 9 g
- Sugar 1.8 g
- Protein 2.3 g
- Cholesterol 0 mg

47-Sausage Meatballs

Preparation Time: 10 minutes
Cooking Time: 15 minutes
Serve: 4

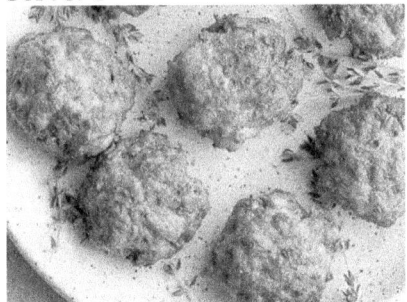

Ingredients:
- 3.5 oz sausage meat
- 3 tbsps almond flour
- 1 tsp ginger garlic paste
- 1/2 onion, diced
- Pepper
- Salt

Directions:
- Preheat the air fryer to 360 F/ 182 C.
- Spray air fryer basket with cooking spray.
- Add all ingredients into the mixing bowl and mix until well combined.
- Make small balls from mixture and place into the air fryer basket and air fry for 15 minutes.
- Serve and enjoy.

Nutritional Value (Amount per Serving):
- Calories 126
- Fat 9.9 g
- Carbohydrates 3.2 g
- Sugar 0.8 g
- Protein 6.4 g
- Cholesterol 21 mg

48-Chicken Meatballs

Preparation Time: 10 minutes
Cooking Time: 10 minutes
Serve: 4

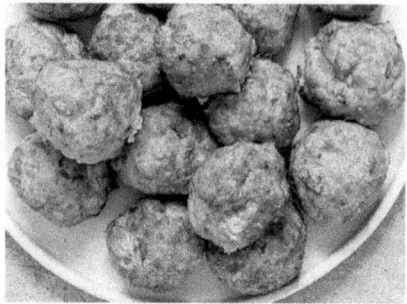

Ingredients:
- 1 lb ground chicken
- 1 tbsp soy sauce
- 1 tbsp hoisin sauce
- 1/2 cup fresh cilantro, chopped
- 1/4 cup shredded coconut
- 1 tsp sesame oil
- 1 tsp sriracha
- 2 green onions, chopped
- Pepper
- Salt

Directions:
- Spray air fryer basket with cooking spray.
- Add all ingredients into the large mixing bowl and mix until well combined.
- Make small balls from mixture and place into the air fryer basket.
- Air fry at 350 F/ 176 C for 10 minutes. Turn halfway through.
- Serve and enjoy.

Nutritional Value (Amount per Serving):
- Calories 258
- Fat 11.4 g
- Carbohydrates 3.7 g
- Sugar 1.7 g
- Protein 33.5 g
- Cholesterol 101 mg

49-Delicious Chicken Kebabs

Preparation Time: 10 minutes
Cooking Time: 6 minutes
Serve: 3

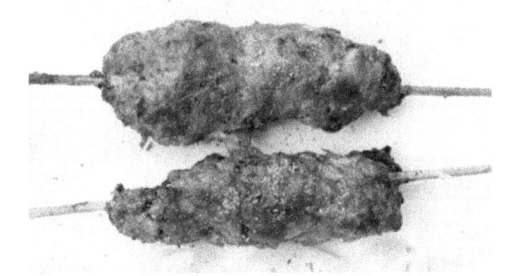

Ingredients:
- 1 lb chicken mince
- 1/4 tsp turmeric powder
- 1 egg, lightly beaten
- 1/3 cup fresh parsley, chopped
- 2 garlic cloves
- 4 oz onion, chopped
- 1/2 tsp black pepper
- 1 tbsp fresh lemon juice
- 1/4 cup almond flour
- 2 green onion, chopped

Directions:
- Add all ingredients into the food processor and process until well combined.
- Transfer chicken mixture to the bowl and place in the fridge for 30 minutes.
- Divide mixture into the six equal portions and roll around the soaked wooden skewers.
- Spray air fryer basket with cooking spray.
- Place kebab skewers into the air fryer basket and air fry at 400 F/200 C for 6 minutes.
- Serve and enjoy.

Nutritional Value (Amount per Serving):
- Calories 329
- Fat 10.9 g
- Carbohydrates 7.9 g
- Sugar 2.5 g
- Protein 48.7 g
- Cholesterol 171 mg

50-Easy Chinese Chicken Wings

Preparation Time: 5 minutes
Cooking Time: 30 minutes
Serve: 2

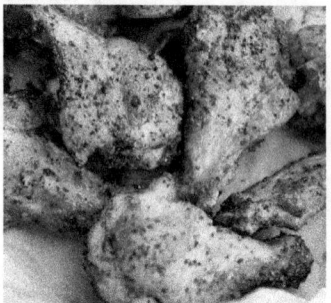

Ingredients:
- 4 chicken wings
- 1 tsp mixed spice
- 1 tbsp soy sauce
- 1 tbsp Chinese spice
- Pepper
- Salt

Directions:
- Add chicken wings into the bowl.
- Add remaining ingredients and toss well.
- Transfer chicken wings into the air fryer basket.
- Air fry at 350 F/ 176 C for 15 minutes.
- Turn chicken to other side and cook for 15 minutes more.
- Serve and enjoy.

Nutritional Value (Amount per Serving):
- Calories 260
- Fat 18.3 g
- Carbohydrates 0.5 g
- Sugar 0.1 g
- Protein 22.1 g
- Cholesterol 0 mg